Alkaline Diet 101

The Complete Alkaline Diet Cookbook for Beginners

Project Vegan

Table of Contents

What is an Alkaline Diet?

The alkaline diet – also known as the alkaline acid diet, alkaline ash diet and even sometimes the pH diet – aids in balancing the pH level of your body's fluids. Your pH is partly defined by the minerals in the foods you eat. To achieve a balance in the body's pH levels, the alkaline diet focuses on foods that are highly alkalinized (certain, non-hybrid fruits and veggies) and removes or limits foods that are acidic (meat and dairy).

It doesn't need to be confusing – you can even drink liquids that can help balance your body's pH levels. For example, **Alkaline water** has a higher pH level than normal drinking water. As such, advocates of the diet recommend that this can be a necessary part of generating the minerals your body requires to begin strengthening symmetry.

Your pH can fall anywhere between 7.35 to 7.45 depending on your diet, the time of day, what you consumed last and when you last used the bathroom. If you frequently consume too many acidic foods, you may develop electrolyte imbalances, and your body's unsteady pH levels can result in too much acidosis. Our bodies find incredible ways of maintaining safe pH levels.

Your body is always going through constant battles in order to maintain this. One way is via your breathing system; the CO_2 you breathe out a few times each minute eliminates the body's acid, which is why it is impossible to hold our breath for a long time without passing out – the rise in acidity will very quickly augment your blood vessels and produce internal imbalances that make alertness impossible.

A healthy, balanced pH environment inside the body can generate health benefits including a stronger immune system, stronger bones and boost heart health. When our body digests the food we eat, it actually burns the foods in a gradual and precise fashion. Once this takes place, the foods leave powder ash that may be acidic, alkaline or neutral. Depending on the proportions of the diet, this ash can either improve or hinder your health, with acid ash leaving you more prone to disease while alkaline ash protects health, and neutral ash has barely any effect.

Live well and take care of your body and health by nourishing and feeding it with nutrients. Our body distributes pH with our kidneys and lungs, and by making sure these two organs stay healthy, we can help our bodies get rid of any excess acid and flourish.

Like all other organs, the kidneys flourish on a simple ensemble of minerals. Chloride, magnesium, and potassium are the three main minerals that allow our kidneys to function at their best, and – sadly – are mildly found in the modern diet.

The Standard American Diet (SAD) consists of many highly-processed carbohydrates, sugary drinks, and animal proteins high in saturated fats. These foods make it harder for the body to digest vitamins and nutrients and provide very little health benefits. They hinder the kidneys and the body altogether. The good news is that establishing a diet that's based on alkalinity is rather easy to do. Foods that are rich in the nutrition and minerals the kidneys, lungs and organs flourish on including fresh fruits, leafy green vegetables, and plant-based protein sources.

By choosing a nutrient-rich Alkaline diet, you can provide your kidneys and lungs with the body's ideal pH of just around 7.4. These can seem like small benefits, but they can bring big results!

How to Eat an Alkaline Diet

Whenever available, shop for organic alkaline foods. And ideally, you will want to learn about the type of compost your produce was grown in — since fruits and vegetables grown in mineral-dense, organic compost tend to be higher in alkaline. Studies have shown that the kind of compost that foods are grown in can drastically affect their vitamin and mineral content, which means that not all alkaline foods are the same.

The proper pH of compost for the optimal overall availability of nutrients in foods is between 6 and 7. Acidic compost below a pH of 6 may have lower calcium and magnesium, and compost higher than a pH of 7 may deplete chemicals such as iron, copper, manganese and zinc. Compost that's finely-incorporated, organically kept and open to wildlife/cattle grazing is usually the healthiest.

If you're curious to figure out your pH level before applying the tips below, you can purchase strips at your local pharmacy store and run simple tests yourself. You can calculate your pH through your saliva or urine. Your first few morning urinations will give you the most accurate results. You contrast the colors on your pH strip to the chart in your test kit. During the day, the ideal time to do a pH test is an hour prior to a meal and two hours after a meal. As for testing saliva, you want to remain between 6.8 and 7.2.

What is pH?

The term pH, which is an <u>acronym</u> for "potential for hydrogen," originated in 1090 by Danish biochemist Søren Lauritz Sørensen. pH is used to specify the quantity of hydrogen ions in a fluid. A hydrogen ion is a basic charged particle, a proton aligned with the symbol H+.

The amount of free hydrogen ions determines the grade of its acidity and the higher the quantity of hydrogen ions that are active, the more acidic your body becomes. By displaying the amount of hydrogen ions, pH indicates whether a fluid is alkaline, acidic, or neutral.

The pH scale

An important thing to take into consideration is that pH values are defined by the concentration of hydrogen ions known as moles (or molecular weight) per liter.

Pure water is a neutral element and has a quantity of hydrogen ions that is equivalent to 0.0000001, or 10^{-7} moles per liter. In contrast, highly acidic substances can contain hydrogen ion concentrations anywhere between 0.01, or 10^{-2} moles per liter.

As these examples show, the amount of hydrogen ions in a substance is defined as a power of 10. To indicate the substance's pH value, we eliminate the base number 10 as well as the minus sign. As a result, a pH of 7 is the rate of pure (neutral) water; a pH of 2 implies high acidity, and a pH of 12 implies high alkalinity.

A boost of a single point of pH is equal to a ten-times reduction in hydrogen ion consolidation. At the same time, a reduction of a single point of pH equals a ten-times increase in hydrogen ion consolidation. If we comprehend this, we can conclude that slight changes in the pH range signify a big change in acid consolidation.

Top Alkaline Foods and Drinks

Wandering the aisles of your local grocery store has turned into some sort of quasi-obstacle course, where processed foods, refined sugars, saturated and trans-fats, and unpronounceable chemicals are singing out to invade your shopping basket. But in a society that prioritizes convenience, it can be challenging to pick out what foods are actually good for you. In addition, there are various diet regimens and rules circulating that will have you wondering if you are actually making the right choice.

Grocery shopping should not be this complicated. The purpose of food and drinks are to fuel the body and help it perform better. However, too many of the ingredients in today's readily available foods are loaded with harmful, acidic ingredients that are detrimental to our body's natural course. Acid-producing foods cause a surplus of acid to form in the body which leads to acidosis.

A good rule of thumb is to search for primarily, fresh, unpackaged foods with ingredients you are familiar with. Below, we will provide a list of the best alkaline foods and drinks that are necessary to succeed in an alkaline diet.

100 Best Alkaline Foods

Spinach

Spinach is loaded with essential vitamins and minerals, and the most alkalinizing food on our list. It's low in cholesterol and saturated fats and is a great source of dietary fiber, protein, and Vitamin A, C, E, and K. Not convinced yet? It's rich in riboflavin, thiamin, folate, calcium, iron, magnesium and Vitamin B6. (All alkaline-generating minerals!) Research also shows that spinach is a potent antioxidant and helps to prevent various different cancers.

Kale

Sharing many of the benefits to its leafy counterpart, kale has a handful of incredible nutritional benefits – and is highly alkalizing. A small cup of kale comprises more than 200% of your Daily Vitamin A Value as well as 130% of Vitamin C and a remarkable 684% of Vitamin K!

There's no possibility of anyone getting grossed out with this powerhouse vegetable in your diet. Loaded with enzyme sulforaphane, kale helps in fighting cancer and other illnesses. Kale is a great addition to salads, soups, smoothies – and my personal favorite snack – chips!

Cucumbers

While cucumbers are not as popular as their "superfood" friends, this largely farmed cultivated vegetable offers a particular combination of vitamins and minerals that allow your body to easily neutralize acidity and maintain alkalinity. Cucumbers are an excellent source of antioxidants as they are made up of phytonutrients such as lignans, cucurbitacins, and flavonoids. These phytonutrients also contain anti-cancer and anti-inflammatory benefits. Not only are they loaded with these incredible nutrients, but they also consist of mostly water – so there is little to no chance you will suffer from dehydration.

Our favorite way of eating these deductible gourds is to simply cut them into thin strips and dip them in a nutritious paste like hummus or tzatziki, or as an addition to sandwiches and salads.

Broccoli

A nutritional powerhouse packed with potassium, Vitamin C and Vitamin K, a great addition to any dish – broccoli is also made up of various other minerals in lesser amounts such as iron, folate and manganese – which all help your body neutralize dangerous acidity. An important component of broccoli, sulforaphane has safeguarding effects against many types of cancer according to the NCBI.

Beyond the previously mentioned health benefits, broccoli can also help lower cholesterol levels and improve eye health. We like chopping them up in halves and eating them with hummus as a snack, but the sky is the limit in terms of what variety you want to choose.

Avocado

Avocados are a highly nutritious and alkaline fruit that have an array of health benefits. While it might be seen as a comfort food due to its fat content, it's actually a fantastic source of fatty acids like oleic acid which has been found to help prevent heart disease and inflammation and heart disease according to the NCBI.

Celery

Yes, it's a fact that celery has more uses than just a base for your soup or a topping for your weekend salad. The health benefits of celery start with its beneficial enzymes and antioxidant properties. It also contains essential vitamins and minerals including Vitamin C, Vitamin K, Vitamin B6, potassium and folate. The most important part of celery, however, is its high water content and tremendous fiber content that improves digestion and weight loss.

Celery is not only highly alkalizing, but also one of the most calorically dilute foods in the world – so snack away! A childhood favorite is "Ants on a Log" which is celery, layered with peanut butter and raisins (an unusual combo – but absolutely delicious).

Sprouts

Although not many studies have been conducted on sprouts in comparison to other vegetables, they are still a source of many nutritional benefits. These little guys provide you with an array of vitamins and minerals with every bite. Sprouts like alfalfa are rich in potassium, magnesium, calcium, iron and zinc – which all fight to neutralize acidity and regenerate your body's mineral deposits.

Sunflower and radish sprouts contain chlorophyll, which has been linked to helping prevent cancer according to studies published by the NCBI. A popular way of enjoying sprouts is by topping them on salads or adding them to sandwiches for a satisfying and delicious crunch.

Other Foods to Consider in an Alkaline Diet

In addition to the foods above, there are many other alkaline foods that nourish the body with rich doses of alkalinizing vitamins and minerals. Here is a list below!

Alkalizing Vegetables

- Alfalfas
- Arugula/Rocket
- Artichokes
- Asparagus
- Baby potatoes
- Barley grass
- Beets
- Brussels sprouts
- Sea vegetables (kelp, dulse, etc.)
- Capsicum/Peppers
- Cabbage
- Carrots
- Chives
- Collards

- Dandelions
- Endives
- Eggplants
- Garlic
- Green beans
- Green peas
- Leeks
- Lettuce
- Mustard greens
- Mushrooms
- Onion
- Parsnips
- Radishes
- Red onions
- Peas
- Pumpkins
- Rhubarb
- Rutabaga
- Sweet potatoes
- Watercress
- Zucchini

Alkalizing Fruit

- Apples
- Apricots
- Bananas
- Blueberries
- Blackberries
- Cranberries
- Fresh coconut (meat and water)
- Fresh dates
- Grapes
- Honeydew Melon
- Limes
- Mangos
- Nectarines
- Oranges
- Peaches
- Pineapples
- Tangerines
- Tomatos
- Strawberries
- Sweet cherries

Alkalizing Nuts & Seeds

- Almonds
- Brazil nuts
- Chestnuts
- Chia seeds
- Flax seeds
- Hemp seeds
- Hazel nuts
- Pecan nuts
- Pumpkin seeds
- Sunflower seeds

Alkalizing Green Powders

- Chlorella
- Spirulina

Alkalizing Spices & Herbs

- Basil
- Cilantro
- Cinnamon
- Dill
- Ginger
- Oregano

- Thyme
- Turmeric

Alkalizing Grains & Beans

*Be sure to soak and sprout before using

- Black beans
- Buckwheat 90
- Butter beans
- Chickpeas
- Lentils
- Millet
- Mung beans
- Navy beans
- Quinoa
- Oats
- White beans
- Wild rice

Best Alkaline Drinks

Almond Milk

Be cautious when roaming the aisles because not all almond milk is good for your health. Keep an eye out for brands that use artificial sweeteners or sugar and instead go for a more natural, unsweetened variety.

The best part about this delectable elixir? It's readily available at most major brand coffee shops. Substitute whole milk for almond milk for a delicious and alkalinizing morning latte.

Juice

No matter where you live, chances are a great variety of juices are readily available almost everywhere – from the gas station to the checkout at the grocery store to your favorite brunch spot. But as stated earlier, not all juices are created equal.

When looking for a good option, choose the brand with the most vegetables per serving. Avoid bottles that include added sugar or artificial sweeteners – any good quality fruit and vegetable juice should be able to satisfy your cravings without any flavor enhancers. Our recommendation? Make your own home-made juice; that way you know exactly what it's made out of.

Lemonade

Before you go down to your local neighborhood lemonade stand, hear us out first. Traditional lemonade is loaded with sugar; an equally refreshing alternative is alkaline water with lemon juice. Lemons are an amazing source of potassium and folate and a great source of Vitamin C. So, pick up a cold glass of alkaline water, squeeze a slice of lemon, and enjoy some sunshine with your *healthy* lemonade.

Coconut Water

Say goodbye to acidic sport drinks with artificial sweeteners and say hello to nature's own sports drink – coconut water. Loaded with Vitamin C, calcium, riboflavin and dietary fiber, this refreshing drink will not only quench your thirst after an intense workout, but it also nourishes your body. Packed with electrolytes, this drink is excellent for workout recovery.

When buying pre-packaged, look out for brands that use artificial flavors or sugars as sweeteners. Look for options with the smallest ingredient list, so you know you are getting the most natural variety available.

Herbal tea

Herbal tea is not only suitable for those gloomy, winter days – it's great for any season or occasion. With various flavors to choose from, this alkaline and delicious drink can be consumed iced or hot. For an extra health boost, try adding fresh sliced ginger to your hot tea or water. Ginger is helpful in relieving stomach problems, loss of appetite, motion sickness and nausea.

Alkaline Water

Last but not least is the healthiest (and simplest) alkaline drink on the market, mineralized alkaline water. Head over to your local supermarket and choose from a variety of brands such as Essentia, PHure, LIFEWTR and Real Water. Say goodbye to hazardous heavy metals and disinfectants and hello to crystal clear alkalinized water that will aid your body in maintaining a healthy pH and lead to improved overall health.

Action Plan

Now that you have a good idea of what to look out for as you stroll down your local grocery store aisle and how to cook these foods once you bring them home, it's time to create an action plan. If your goal is to neutralize acidity enough to stay alkaline, it is not mandatory to eliminate all acidic foods at once. In fact, a successful healthy, alkaline diet is about maintaining balance.

Ideally, you would like to follow an 80/20 Alkaline Diet rule; which means consuming 80% alkaline foods and drinks and only 20% acidic foods and drinks. Most people don't feel pressured to eliminate many foods because enjoying a good snack here and there is still healthy. You don't have to shun your favorite Starbucks espresso or occasional bag of chips completely, but you should base your diet around fresh fruits and vegetables.

Avoid a Massive Reliance on Processed Foods

The world we live in is a fast-paced one; we are always on-the-go, so we tend to take priority on choosing convenience over quality most of the time. This puts our diets in a quality that the nutrition provided by whole foods. So to get you back on track, here are some simple guidelines to make sure you transition to a whole foods vegan diet in a simple layout.

Pretend Processed Foods Do Not Exist

This may sound too intense, but don't be discouraged just yet. Imagine rummaging through the store and not finding any pre-packaged food to choose from, like frozen meals, cereals, or boxed dinners. Not a single processed granola bar or any food with a lengthy list of ingredients. Now, if these options were not available to you, you would not have a choice but to buy the healthier foods.,

I am not saying that you should steer away from everything you find packaged or boxed. Foods like hummus, whole grains, protein bars, ground flax or chia, nut butter, salsa, seaweed snacks, frozen veggies, kale chips, frozen fruits, and even non-dairy milk are all completely tolerable (not all of them are inexpensive, though.) The goal is to eat mostly foods that contain five or fewer ingredients. If you have decided to keep buying prepared foods. Just keep away from those that have overt oils .

Plan Your Meals

It is important to prepare your meals at least a week in advance, after all exercise is not the only aspect of achieving great health. Keep your meals and snacks ready to go anytime you want. This keeps you away from reaching for unhealthy pre-packaged choices any time it's convenient.

If you are short on time. How about using your lunch break a couple of days a week to stock up on healthy food supplies? Or if that's not enough time, just take a look at your schedule and try to crowbar in some opportunities to do your meal prepping chores. If all this fails, you can always hire a professional meal prepper from sites like www.snagajob.com sure it may be expensive, but if you value your time delegating to a freelancer is well worth the money.

The bottom line on processed foods

Think of processed foods not precisely as an addiction, but as a set back to your health almost just as much as drugs, alcohol, and tobacco. Always choose wisely what you eat, and even more so before and after a workout and you will find that you performance at the gym will improve immensely, and overall you will improve your health.

The Importance of Whole Foods and Color Variety

So as to carry out a plant-based diet properly, consume foods that are the least deviated from their natural state as possible. A broad range of whole plant foods in as many colors as you can will ensure you are attaining lots of rich minerals, vitamins, antioxidants, amino acids, proteins, and phytonutrients. Consumption of colorful foods like vegetables, dark-colored fruits, green tea, and berries can aid in the reduction of disease probability, quick recovery and safeguard cellular health.

A great place to begin is consuming a broad range of vegetables. I always suggest consumption of one large raw salad daily. It can be loaded up with as many vegetables as you prefer, then a few healthy fats like avocado and hemp seed can be added, also add a little protein like edamame or lentils if required, then it can be topped using apple cider vinegar or fat-free dressing.

Use the five-ingredient rule

If there is an excess of five ingredients on a nutrition label, it is a clear sign of an overtly processed food, try to avoid these. This will be the easiest and most straight forward way of preventing impulse buying on most unhealthy processed foods.

Stick to whole grains

Whole grain pasta, whole grain cereal and, whole grain bread – you get the idea. Eliminating carbs is unnecessary, in fact, you should embrace them as they are fundamental to a healthy vegan diet; Eating a clean diet simply means having an understanding of which carbs the best for you. Whole grain is always a safe bet.

Revamp your Food Environment

It might be time to clear out your cupboards. One great way to ensure you don't consume junk food is to keep it out of your home altogether. Like most addictions, the best way to get it out of your life is to nip it in the bud.

You can't eat junk food if it is not there, and when it is an inconvenience to go to the store for a late night snack, you will ask yourself if it is worth the effort. Once you create a healthy food environment you will grow accustomed to loving the foods you are surrounded by.

Mistakes Happen

Most changes are difficult, and letting go of unhealthy addictive food is a tough change for most people. If once in a while you give in and eat junk foods, don't blame yourself and give up. After all, we are human and this is a transitional process, we can always turn a mistake into a learning opportunity. Remember you do not need to be perfect to succeed, and strive to make whole foods the main part of your diet slowly but surely.

Anti-inflammatory foods

Around 12.9 million people around the world have lost their lives due to some cardiovascular disease, according to statistics from the World Health Organization in 2012. It is estimated that each year, about eight million people lose their lives to cancer. Cancer and heart disease are expected to remain as the primary cause of death in developed countries following a western diet for many years to come.

To increase your odds of preventing these common health hazards, it's recommended to add anti-inflammatory foods to your diet. Below we have a list of the recommended foods that are essential inflammatory preventers.

What is Acidosis?

When the fluids in your body become too acidic, it transforms into a substance known as acidosis. Acidosis is the result of your kidney and lungs not being able to maintain your body's pH in check. Much of the body's functions generate acid. Your kidneys and lungs can usually recompense for minor pH imbalances,

The blood in your body's acidity can be measured by calculating its pH. A diminished pH means that you have highly acidic blood while a elevated pH means that your blood is stable. According to the American Association for Clinical Chemistry (AACC) your blood's pH should ideally be around 7.4. acidosis is defined by a pH of 7.35 or less. Alkalosis is defined by a pH level of 7.45 or more.

While seemingly low, these numerical distinctions can be severe. Acidosis can result in a large quantity of health issues and can even be a giant health risk.

Causes of acidosis

There are two versions of acidosis, and both have unique causes. The acidosis type is defined as either metabolic acidosis or respiratory acidosis, altering based on the main cause of your acidosis.

Respiratory acidosis

Repertory acidosis is a result of too much C02 building up in the body. Typically, the lungs disperse CO_2 when you breathe. However, occasionally, your body is not able to eliminate enough CO_2. This usually happens due to:

- asthma and other airway conditions
- chest injuries
- obesity, which makes breathing more difficult
- excessive alcohol
- muscle frailty in the chest
- complications with the nervous system
- malformed chest structure

Metabolic acidosis

Metabolic acidosis begins in the kidneys rather than the lungs. It happens when they are not able to eliminate enough acid or when they cut off too much base.

Diabetic acidosis

Diabetic acidosis develops in people with diabetes that is badly contained. If your body does not have enough insulin, ketones form in your body and acidify your blood.

Hyperchloremic acidosis

Hyperchloremic acidosis occurs from a deficiency of sodium bicarbonate. This base is crucial in keeping your blood neutral. Both vomiting and diarrhea can cause this type of acidosis.

Lactic acidosis

Lactic acidosis develops when there's an excess of lactic acid in your body. Root causes can include cancer, chronic alcohol use, heart failure, seizures, liver failure and low blood sugar.

Renal tubular acidosis

Renal tubular acidosis develops if the kidneys cannot excrete acids into the urine. This makes the blood more acidic.

How Acidic Foods Affect the Body

Acidic blood is linked to severe health conditions, such as kidney stones, a higher risk of concern (a high acidic environment is ideal for the growth of cancer cells) and can even impede the liver from being able to detoxify properly.

Bone density can also be hindered by acidic blood. This is due to calcium (and alkaline mineral) being extracted from the bones to nullify the blood's pH when it starts to become too acidic.

Many people experience stomach ache from eating too many acidic foods – but regardless of acidifying foods, the cause depends on an individual's environment and overall health.

The stomach lining naturally fights off acidity as stomach acids naturally consume stomach acid. But in many cases, people who have digestive problems like stomach ulcers or acid reflux might be distressed by acidic foods.

Foods that are not acidic but contain acidifying minerals before digestion can sometimes agitate existing digestive problems as their acidity (not their pH) can take effect prior to digestion.

A surplus of acidity may become a hazard that weakens all body functions and is a very common health condition. It aids an internal environment ideal for diseases, as opposed to a pH balanced environment which permits the normal body function required for it to combat disease. A healthy body preserves sufficient alkaline stores to meet emergency demands. When too much acid needs to be neutralized, our alkaline stores are reduced resulting in a weaker body.

Most people who don't have a blanked pH are acidic. This condition makes the body borrow minerals— including calcium, magnesium, sodium and potassium—from vital bones and organs to neutralize the acid and properly extract it from the body.

Due to this strain, the body can experience severe and drawn-out damage due to excessive acidity—a condition that might go undiscovered for years. Mild acidosis can cause problems such as:

- Cardiovascular damage, which expands the blood vessels and depletes oxygen.

- Weight gain and diabetes which results in bladder and kidney problems such as kidney stones.

- Acceleration of radical damage, possibly assisting the growth of cancerous mutations.

- Osteoporosis which results in weak, frail bones, bone spurs and hip fractures.

- Joint pain, cramping muscles and acid buildup.

- Energy depletion and chronic fatigue.

The human body produces acid, non-stop, every day as an appendage of the metabolism. In addition, acid is passed into the system through consumption and digestion. Many extracted and digested acids are cleared away by the bloodstream and discharged from the body in the urine.

Other acids are released from the body though perspiration. Your body can only absorb a limited amount of acids; however, it can possibly overwhelm the system and cause the body to become acidic.

Acidity is linked to disease:

- Acid reflux is a painful condition that happens when acidic fluid congests (refluxes) into the esophagus resulting in inflammation, irritation and affliction to the lining of the esophagus.

- High cholesterol happens when the body creates a surplus of cholesterol to neutralize the acids in the bloodstream before they harm living cells.

- Heart disease is the outcome of too much cholesterol building up in the coronary arteries that lessens the blood flow to the heart. As mentioned earlier, cholesterol forms to protect the arterial tract from the acidity in the blood.

- Inflammatory related conditions such as arthritis, allergies, fibromyalgia and even stroke are linked to a low-count metabolic acidosis.

A recent seven-year-long study done at the University of San Francisco on 9,000 women concluded that those who suffer from chronic acidosis are at a higher risk of bone-related diseases than those who have balanced pH levels.

The researchers who carried out this stuff believe that a large portion of the hip injuries prevalent among middle-aged women are linked to high acidity induced by a diet high in animal products and low in vegetables. This is the result of the body borrowing calcium from the bones in order to neutralize pH.

Drinking clean alkaline water can help replenish the body's pH balance, lessen acidity and encourage detoxification.

Acidosis & Energy Production

In order for our cells to function properly, they need to be in a balanced state of acid-alkaline. If not, this drastically reduces the cells' ability to create energy via the cellular energy composites known as mitochondria. Stored within the cells, mitochondria are the main producers of a compound known as ATP (adenosine triphosphate) which provides the energy that cells, organs and tissues require to properly function.

Even a minor acidic inclination within the cells creates a defective function of mitochondrial electron passage, resulting in both depleted energy production and increased energy loss. Deficiency of ATP caused by excessive alkaline or acidic pH results in fatigue and can ultimately cause pain and hinder organ function.

To neutralize the cellular issues caused by depleted acidosis, the body's system of homeostasis – its capability to self-adjust and thus manage internal balance among alkali mineral deposits, such as the alkaline salts of calcium, potassium and magnesium. These minerals, which are contained mainly within the musculoskeletal, structure, are absorbed by the body to quench acid growth.

If the variations in acid-alkaline levels are only momentary, homeostasis is typically restored. But if the imbalances continue unaddressed, ultimately the body's ability to control homeostasis is overpowered, resulting in a state of "dis-ease" that will, over time, start to attack the most vulnerable and susceptible organ systems.

Acidosis diminishes available oxygen

Compounding this issue is the factor that acidosis also depletes the quantity of oxygen accessible to the body's cells and tissues. Furthermore, a shortage of oxygen interferes with mitochondrial function and also diminishes the cells' capacity to properly replenish and repair themselves. The low-oxygen climate formed by acidosis also encourages the growth of harmful microorganisms.

This, too, builds fatigue by interrupting the body's ability to properly incorporate and use up the nutrients gathered from food. The culminating nutritional deficiencies not only deplete the creation of enzymes of hormones required for energy production but can hinder consumption of the nutrients gathered from food.

An acidic tilt compromises immunity

The body's immune defense system operates best in a very linear pH range. Acid-alkaline imbalances can hinder the body's capacity to fight off malicious microorganisms such as bacteria, viruses and fungi. The reasons these things happen are many, with two having the most importance to our dialogue.

First, when blood pH inclines towards imbalance, the body's cells are unable to properly receive essential nutrients and oxygen from blood stores. In addition, the cells begin to struggle in disposing of wastes. In both cases, these reactions are the result of diminished permeability of cellular membranes, now hardened by an imbalance in acid-alkaline.

As the cell walls harden, not only are nutrients and oxygen unable to penetrate the cells, but waste is unable to be eliminated. Together, these circumstances lead to weaker cells that are unable to act as nature intended.

The second factor that depletes immunity is the way that acid-alkaline imbalances allow infectious agents to be grown and replicate inside the body. Contrary to popular belief, people do not become ill by simply becoming exposed to infectious pathogens.

The truth is that people are constantly exposed to such microorganisms. In addition, there are thousands of different potentially hazardous bacteria growing within our gastrointestinal tracts every day. Yet, the majority of the time, they are not individually capable of causing illness. This is epitomized during elevated times of infection such as flu season, and although not everyone catches flu or a cold, more people are exposed to the viruses that cause them.

A large factor that decides whether microorganisms can cause sickness is the pH level in the body's interior environment. When the body has a proper acid-alkaline balance, the bloodstream enters an aerobic state— which means that it has a wealthy amount of oxygen. In this circumstance, the body can defend itself from likely hazardous pathogens, as pathogens are not able to thrive in oxygen-rich environments. When acid-alkaline becomes unbalanced and chronic, however, the bloodstream begins to suffer an oxygen deficiency.

This reduced oxygen state allows microorganisms that previously were a non-threat to become pathogenic (disease-causing), as the body cannot properly eradicate them. Furthermore, a low-oxygen environment is optimal for such microorganisms to re-create rapidly inside the body, making it progressively more challenging for the body's immune system to keep them under control.

Osteoporosis and other problems related to mineral loss

In order to halt a surplus of acid generation, the body might be required to draw upon its alkali mineral deposits. The bones are the body's largest repository of mineral reserves, but mineral deposits are also found in the teeth and other organs. Although frequent periods of mineral extraction from bones, organs, and teeth usually do not lead to health problems, constant mineral extraction, or demineralization – in particular, calcium, potassium and magnesium – can result in severe disorders.

One of the most prevalent of said problems is osteoporosis, a condition of intense bone fragility and elevated low-trauma injury risk. In fact, as of 2019, around 10 million Americans over the age of 50 suffer from osteoporosis, and an additional 33 million Americans are susceptible due to their low bone mass. There is a certain link between chronic low-grade metabolic acidosis and osteoporosis.

A variety of global population-based studies has concluded the link between high consumption of base-forming foods (mostly fruits and veggies) and bone health.

The favorable impact of fruits and veggie consumption on bone mass is noticeable not only in premenopausal and postmenopausal women—those at highest risk of osteoporosis—but also in developing girls and boys.

Additionally, an extensive cross-global survey (Abelow et al. 1992) determined that those countries with the lowest prevalence of hip injuries also have the lowest intake of acid-building animal protein, and typically, an intake of vegetable protein that surpasses their consumption of animal products. Of course, the diet practiced by these cultures is drastically different from the common Western diet, which is loaded with acid-building animal proteins and low in base-building, pH balancing foods.

Unfortunately, severe bone mineral loss can also contribute to other bone debilitating diseases, including osteoarthritis, rheumatism, and degeneration of the disks of the spine. Spine degeneration, as a result, can suffer other problems, such as sciatica and chronic back pain. Furthermore, the long-term depletion of minerals can decrease the health of teeth, making them more sensitive to hot and cold foods, and more brittle.

A lack of minerals also brings about dry skin that cracks easily, itches, and ages prematurely. Other conditions usually associated with chronic mineral loss are thinning of hair, blood loss and overly sensitive gums.

Acidosis & Inflammation

Inflammation is our body's natural reaction to the necessity for repair and is, therefore, fundamental to the healing process. Through the inflammatory period, brittle tissue, or tissue weakened by trauma are dissolved and recycled in preparation for its replacement with new vital tissue. However, the inflammation or tissue depletion becomes severe; the healing process is not completed, and a wide spectrum of possible health issues can arise.

Acidosis creates a rich optimal ground for inflammation in various ways. For example, the elevated levels of dangerous microorganisms induced by acidosis can lead to inflammation.

In addition to this, when organs and tissues are exposed to acids, they start to harden and/or grow lesions in order to defend themselves. As an additional defense mechanism, they may begin to engorge in an attempt to stop acids from penetrating the tissues. These inflammatory responses can happen anywhere in the body but typically start in the organ structures that are fragile as an outcome of genetics or pre-existing health issues.

If inflammation continues, it can ultimately lead to an array of disease conditions, which include arthritis, bronchitis, colitis, neuritis, skin conditions like hives and rashes, and urinary tract disruptions such as painful urination and cystitis (bladder infection). Furthermore, chronic inflammation can decrease immune function-ability which is already depleted due to the generation of unhealthy microorganisms.

Dining Out on the Alkaline Diet

The trend is shifting to whatever customers are demanding about their restaurant food preferences. Here are some tips you might find helpful to manage your alkaline deposits when you are out on the town.

Analyze your restaurant options

Instead of getting recommendations from friends who might not be as health conscious as you, make it your obligation to find one yourself. When looking around, find spots where the food is freshly prepared and as whole food based as possible. Mom and pop diners, ethnic restaurants, and establishments that offer vegan menus are usually alkaline friendly.

Bypass the bread appetizer

Bread is usually served first to "quieten down" ones appetite. However Bread is acidic and not essential so contemplate vegetable soup or a salad as an appetizer instead.

"A-la-carte" orders might be your best choice

Focus on side dish orders and assemble a tasty and healthy meal with an alkalizing vegetable soup or salad and a side dish of baked potatoes and steamed veggies.

Beverage options

A little health consciousness can do wonders when choosing a beverage. Spring water/purified water is usually a good choice and just a few drops of lemon/lime away to being alkaline. Orange or grape juice and water can be mixed for a refreshing drink. Green tea is always a great option. And for a drink that is a great addition to any meal, try some steamed water with a pinch of lemon. This relaxing drink is relaxing, helps digestion, and is highly energizing. Try it you may be pleasantly surprised.

Remember the 80% rule

As nutrition guru Dr. Max Gerson has regularly suggested, if a person eats 80% of their food to be as healthy as possible, then most people can grant the remaining 20% to be more of a "personal or recreational preference" nature.

How to Create an Alkaline Diet Plan

Are you familiar with the alkalinity of the foods you eat? Should you care? It is common knowledge that the food we eat has a great impact on our health and wellbeing, and incorporating whole, alkalinizing foods can help us in feeling our best.

Take Stock of Your Pantry

Since the Alkaline diet is not based on being a perfectionist, keep in mind the 80/20 rule when doing your grocery shopping. Buy plenty of fresh fruits and veggies, nuts and beans while granting yourself 20 percent of acidic non-animal-based foods like processed foods, coffee, and sweeteners.

In order to effectively practice a healthy lifestyle, you might need to do a bit more meal preparation than you are accustomed to. Beginning with an energizing breakfast like acai granola or a spinach and fruit smoothie will assure you have a spike in energy, especially if you choose to eliminate coffee. You can switch your early morning latte with green tea, energizing kombucha and almond milk.

If your weekly habits entail lunch gatherings and dubious menus, you should memorize a few basic substitutes and adjustments to keep on track when eating out. Go with a vegan salad with no dressing, rather than some light vinaigrette. Soups and stews with no animal products, stir-fried vegetables and veggie wraps with quinoa or wild rice are other great options to look out for.

If you would like to optimize your options, pack pre-made lunches and plenty of fresh snacks to keep with you throughout the day, so you are always on track and sated.

Stay Hydrated

When the temperature is high, getting properly hydrated is crucial, regardless if you are physically active or just laying on a sunny beach.

Not drinking a large glass of water before a morning run, sweating excessively during workouts, and withstanding hot temperatures are sure ways to become dehydrated. Consuming water during exercising can also aid in battling fatigue and lengthen your endurance. Below are some ways to determine if you are appropriately hydrated that are easy and convenient to follow.

Urine color

Your urine color can be a good sign. If it is a clean water color, then the likelihood that you are hydrated is very high. If the color is dark or has a strange odor, that is an indicator that you are dehydrated. Please note that if you are consuming a B12 supplement, it can have an impact on your urine color, but it does not mean you are dehydrated, but always check with your doctor to be sure what is going on if you are suspicious of anything.

Rate of sweat

Another method to determine your hydration level is to check your weight before and after working out. The before/after hydrating weight difference will provide you a sign of your hydration level. If you have added or kept the same weight, you could conclude that you're hydrated. If you are down in weight by a noticeable amount, you will need to drink more water to restore the weight you have lost.

What's the amount of water you should be drinking?

The amount of water you should take differs; a person who sweats significantly should drink higher amounts than someone who doesn't. This is specifically true for athletes who train during hot summer months. For every pound of sweat lost, that's a pint of water you will have to recuperate, which is why it is not strange for a high school football player with pads and running drills to drop five pounds of sweat while practicing during the summer.

Create a hydration habit

Some people work so hard to the point where they hardly have any time to eat, or even catch a regular water break. But making a habit of being hydrated will aid you in maintaining your energy and attention so your body and mind function optimally. Below are some tips to get your fluid fix throughout the day much easier

Always have water on hand, even if you are at work

If you keep a bottle of water near you, it will make it more convenient to sip water throughout the day, without it seeming like a drag. If you start to feel nauseous or fatigued, drink some cold water. It's a quick way to make you more alert anytime you are in a slump.

Mix it up

Does water seem boring? Here are some tips on how you can get other sources of water.

Fuse it

Cut fruit slices, such as lime, oranges, and lemon in a water container and let refrigerate for a few hours.

Add coconut ice cubes

Add the coconut water to your ice cube tray, then scoop the ice cubes in a glass of water for a sweet and nutty taste.

Sip herbal tea

Try sipping on a cup of herbal tea every day. If you do this regularly, you'll have the additional fluids of 1 cup of water to your tally every day. Moreover, this can be a therapeutic way to let go of stress at the day's end.

Eat your water

Try eating these foods for a delicious and simple way of increasing your H20 absorption without directly drinking water.

Not sweating during hardcore exercise can be a sign that you are hydrated to the point of exhaustion due to the heat. Also, you should be careful of sugary drinks or fruit juices and soda, as they can be harsh on your stomach if you are not hydrated. It's also advisable to stay away from drinks that are made up of caffeine, which can perform as a diuretic and result in the loss of more fluids.

Now that you understand the impact hydration can have on you, remember you will not have to worry if you drink at least 11 cups a day as part of your daily habit.

How to Make the Transition

It can feel insanely overwhelming when you're just starting to go vegan. It is a drastic change in lifestyle compared to having the convenience of being able to eat almost anything as an omnivore, especially for people who enjoyed and are used to eating meat and animal products their whole lives. It might even feel almost impossible. Below, we will go over some tips, so you do not get overwhelmed or be too hard on yourself in your transition.

Don't expect perfection

You can expect that you will slip on a vegan diet, regardless if you have or have not yet. After all, we are human. And it's not just our mindset; it's also our body adjusting, from your palate to everything inside your body. My advice is, don't dwell on the times you slipped up, but focus on all the good and healthy choices you've made outside of that one mistake. Remember, it will take more than one slip up to take away all the progress you've made.

Every day as a vegan will reduce your cravings, and you will gradually move towards more healthy food. You will be amazed by how your palate adapts when given the chance.

Specify your start date; the sooner you start the better

When you decide to start, empty your refrigerator of all the meat and animal products, including dairy, fats (like butter) and eggs. Then do the same for your pantry and throw out all the canned or boxed goods that have meat or animal products. You'll want to do this all at the same time. Say your goodbyes to the whole unhealthy lot. Toss them or give them to the local food shelter.

Then get a vegan cookbook (see recommendations below). Or get online where there are many resources for unique and creative vegan meals. You will find that veganism is very visible as long as you look for opportunities.

Draw up a meal plan for your first month to include all the meals you'll have each day: breakfast, lunch, dinner, and snacks. And with this new meal plan, you can now create your grocery list and source your foods for the week.

Eating Cheat Meals and Staying Healthy!

You can enjoy your guilty pleasures and still lose weight. As incredible as it sounds, there is a strategic way to go about this.

Many people create diets that are so strict that they find themselves breaking all the rules in a very short while. It's actually better to new transitioners to loosen up on these rules. It is healthy to indulge once in a while. The key is moderation and making sure the majority of your calories come from healthy whole foods.

Many dieticians have come to a consensus that it is vital to build muscle in "cheat meal days" since depriving yourself of fatty foods can actually lead to increased cravings, causing you to fail on your diet. Additionally, setting your diet aside occasionally stimulates the thyroid gland and can "re-charge" your metabolism.

What you can eat

As stated earlier, you should avoid processed foods on the days you have set aside as your cheat days. This means you should avoid chips and any other packaged treats from the snack aisle at the grocery store. For clarity, you can have vegan hamburgers, doughnuts, and cookies. But as a rule, do not eat them in their processed forms. For the best results, your cheat meals should be your favorite homemade delicacies.

In conclusion, you can permit cheat meals as a means of aiding your dieting process, and this is the plan you have created and adjusted to for losing weight and becoming healthier. Cheat meals become a problem when you start eating them without any control all through the day. The ideal time for a cheat meal should not exceed 30 to 40 minutes. It is a tough path to follow, but the benefits at the end of your journey are worth it. Your cheat meals will add value to your entire dieting plan if you adhere to the rules of satisfying your cravings moderately.

What is the best time to eat a cheat meal?

While the purpose of cheat meals is to satiate your urge for junk foods, they still need to be eaten in strict moderation. Think of cheat meals as a moment to indulge in "bad" carbs, fats and proteins. For some people, that means switching from complex carbs to simple carbs or adding extra guac to that vegan burrito. Also, always eat your cheat meal after a workout when your body can best absorb both "good" and "bad" macros.

Plan around special occasions

Birthdays, weddings and other gatherings and celebrations are notoriously harsh for people sitting on the sidelines watching others eat. Because of this, it is advisable to schedule your cheat meal for the exact day of a special event, in case it is coming up. However, try to stick to that one meal only, as opposed to other people at the gathering who might adopt an all-you-can-eat mentality.

Let go of the perfectionist streak

When you are indulging in cheat meals, you must seize the opportunity and enjoy it. Many people might even feel guilty after eating a cheat meal, no matter how prepared they were or how well they planned it out.

Most people fail at diet because their expectations are too high and go all in or nothing. It's impossible to always be perfect, so it is best to nip the perfectionist mentality in the bud for the sake of your health in the long run.

Sample 7-Day Alkaline Meal Plan

Assembling a meal plan is the best way to make sure you start off on the right foot and obtain optimal results on this new diet. Here is a basic menu to get your creative juices flowing. Keep in mind that completely eliminating acidic foods is not required for the alkaline diet, so be as flexible as you want as long as you are following an 80/20 rule as mentioned earlier. You can choose to gradually increase the amount of alkalizing foods you eat until you achieve your desired results.

Day One

Breakfast: Strawberry Coco Chia Quinoa

Ingredients:

1 cup quinoa

½ cup quartered strawberries + 3 diced strawberries

5 tablespoons chia seeds

1 ½ cups hemp or coconut milk

2 Medjool pitted dates

2 tablespoons almond chunks

2 tablespoons coconut flakes

Directions:

Overnight, cook the quinoa and strawberry chia by mixing almond milk, strawberries, and 2 dates in a mixer and pulsing until smooth. Pour the mix into a jar and garnish with chia seeds. Mix until the chia seeds are coated with the liquid. Cover and place in the fridge overnight. In the morning, add all ingredients to a bowl and serve cold!

Lunch: Sweet and Savory Salad

Ingredients:

1 head of butter lettuce

1 sliced avocado

¼ cup chopped pistachio meat

½ sliced cucumber

1 seeded pomegranate, or 1/3 cup seeds

Dressing Ingredients:

½ cup olive oil

¼ cup apple cider vinegar

1 minced garlic clove

Directions:

Shred or tear the lettuce into a large bowl. Put in the rest of the ingredients and toss with a tong. Drizzle with salad dressing.

Day Two

Breakfast: Non-Dairy Apple Parfait

Ingredients:

½ cup almond or coconut milk

½ cup soaked cashews (soak 30 minutes - 1 hour)

1 cup diced apple

½ teaspoon vanilla

1/3 cup raw rolled oats

1 tablespoon hemp seeds

Directions:

Mix the milk, cashews and vanilla in a mixer and pulse until smooth. Stack all ingredients in a small cup: Smack a large spoon of cashew cream. Handful of apples, garnish with hemp seeds and oats and enjoy!

Lunch: Savory Avocado Wrap

Ingredients:

1 butter lettuce

½ avocado

Handful of spinach

1 teaspoon minced basil

1 teaspoon chopped cilantro

1 sliced tomato

¼ diced onion

Sea salt & pepper

Directions:

Spread avocado onto a big lettuce leaf and garnish with basil, onion, cilantro, tomato, spinach and add salt and pepper. Fold like tacos and enjoy!

Day Three

Breakfast: Almond Butter Crunchy Berry Smoothie

Ingredients:

2 cups almond milk

2 cups fresh spinach

1 cup of any frozen mixed berries or strawberries

1 banana (skinned and frozen)

4 tablespoons raw almond butter

1 tablespoon chia

Directions:

Blend almond milk and spinach first. Add the rest of the ingredients minus the chia and blend again. Add the chia once the mixture is smooth – then pulse on a low speed to mix. Finally, coat the mixture thoroughly with chia seeds to expand. Enjoy!

Lunch: Kale Pesto Pasta

Ingredients:

2 cups fresh basil

1 handful kale

1/2 cup walnuts

¼ cup extra virgin olive oil

Sea salt and pepper

Juice of 2 limes

1 spiralized zucchini (noodles)

Optional: top with chopped asparagus, tomato and spinach leaves

Directions:

Overnight, soak walnuts to soften. Add all ingredients into a blender, and pulse until the consistency becomes creamy. Add in zucchini noodles and serve!

Day Four

Breakfast: Apple and Almond Butter Oats

Ingredients:

2 cups rolled oats

1 cup finely minced or grated green apple

1 teaspoon cinnamon

1/3 cup raw almond butter

1 ½ cups coconut milk

Directions:

Add the oats, almond butter and coconut milk into a bowl and stir well.

Mix in the grated apple pieces: cover the bowl with a plastic wrap or lid and put in the fridge. Refrigerate overnight. Top off with cinnamon powder and serve.

Lunch: Avocado Salad with Cumin Dressing

Ingredients for dressing:

1 avocado

1 tablespoon cumin powder

¼ teaspoon sea salt

1 tablespoon extra-virgin olive oil

1 cup water

2 squeezed limes

Dash of cayenne pepper

Ingredients for Tahini Lemon Dressing:

¼ cup tahini

1 clove garlic

¾ teaspoon sea salt

½ cup water

½ squeezed lemon

1 tablespoon extra-virgin olive oil

Black pepper

Ingredients for salad:

3 cups chopped kale

½ cup drained kelp noodles

1/3 cup halved cherry tomatoes

½ cup broccoli florets

½ spiralized zucchini (noodles)

2 tablespoons hemp seeds

Directions:

Steam broccoli and kale for 4 minutes and set aside. Add in zucchini and kelp noodles and mix in a heaping serving of the dressing. Add cherry tomatoes and garnish with hemp seeds.

Day Five

Breakfast: Berry Delight Spinach Power Smoothie

Ingredients:

2 cups fresh spinach

2 cups almond milk

1 cup frozen berries (any variety)

1 frozen banana

1 tablespoon coconut oil

½ teaspoon cinnamon

Blend all ingredients in a food processor or blender until all ingredients are creamy and smooth. Enjoy!

2 tablespoons raw almond butter

Directions:

Blend spinach and almond milk first, then add remaining ingredients and blend.

Lunch: Quinoa Burrito Bowl

Ingredients:

1 cup quinoa (or wild rice)

2 15-oz cans of black beans

2 sliced avocados

4 minced garlic cloves

1 teaspoon cumin

4 sliced green onions (scallions)

2 juiced limes

Small handful of chopped cilantro

Directions:

Cook the quinoa or rice. In a separate pot, cook beans over low heat. Mix in onions, garlic, cumin, lime juice and allow flavors to set in for 10-15 minutes. When quinoa is soft, split into individual bowls. Layer with beans, avocado and cilantro.

Day Six

Breakfast: Quinoa Morning Oatmeal

Ingredients:

2 ½ cups coconut milk

½ cup quinoa

1 teaspoon chia seeds

1 teaspoon hemp seeds

1 teaspoon cinnamon

Directions:

Mix all ingredients except for hemp seeds and cook on low for 10-15 minutes until liquid has evaporated. Garnish with hemp seeds and serve.

Lunch: Thai Quinoa Salad

Ingredients for dressing:

1 tablespoon sesame seeds

1 teaspoon lemon juice

2 teaspoon tamaris

1 teaspoon chopped garlic

3 teaspoons apple cider vinegar

½ teaspoon sea salt

¼ cup tahini (sesame butter)

½ teaspoon toasted sesame oil

1 pitted date

Ingredients for salad:

1 cup of steamed quinoa

1 sliced tomato

1 handful of arugula

¼ diced red onion

Directions:

In a blender, add the following: 2 tablespoons + ¼ cup water, then the remaining ingredients. Blend well. Cook 1 cup of quinoa in a rice cooker or steamer, then let cool down. Mix in the arugula, quinoa, red onion, tomatoes onto a salad bowl, add the Thai dressing, and toss until the salad is fully coated and serve.

Day Seven

Breakfast: Warrior Chia Breakfast

Ingredients:

1 cup almond or coconut milk

4 tablespoons chia seeds

½ teaspoon cinnamon

½ teaspoon vanilla

¼ cup chopped almonds

1 tablespoon coconut flakes

Directions:

Overnight, mix milk and chia seeds in a jar. Add chopped almonds, vanilla, and cinnamon. Cover tightly with a lid and shake the mix until it's combined. Refrigerate overnight. In the morning, pour the mix into two bowls. Garnish with coconut flakes or fresh fruits.

Lunch: Asian Sesame Dressing and Noodles

Ingredients for dressing:

2 teaspoons tamaris

2 tablespoon tahini

½ teaspoon liquid coconut nectar

½ teaspoon lemon juice

1 minced garlic clove

Ingredients for noodle salad:

1 spiralized zucchini (noodles) or a pack of kelp noodles

1 chopped scallion

1 tablespoon raw sesame seeds

Optional: sliced red bell pepper/carrot

Directions:

In a salad bowl, mix all dressing ingredients and stir well with a spoon. Make the zucchini noodles using a spiralizer, or put kelp noodles in warm water for a few minutes so they wash off the liquid they are packaged with. Mix the dressing into the noodles and stir toss thoroughly. Sprinkle with sesame seeds on top and serve.

There you have it. You are now well on your way to weight the Keto Vegan way!

Be prepared to feel great, have energy you never had before and achieve the weight loss results you always desired! Thank you for taking the time to read my book and stay tuned for more books on Veganism in the future.

If you enjoyed my book and would recommend it to anyone. I'd be very grateful if you can leave a short review on Amazon. Your feedback is really important and I will use the opportunity to find out how I can improve this book even more.

Thanks again for your support!

www.ingramcontent.com/pod-product-compliance
Lightning Source LLC
Chambersburg PA
CBHW051359280526
45784CB00007B/3026